W0106352

Preface

During the First European Congress of Anesthesiology, held in Vienna, Austria, in September, 1962, panel discussions on nineteen different subjects were held, each lasting approximately three hours. One, concerning Controversial Aspects of Resuscitation, was later edited by its chairman, PETER SAFAR, and published in 1963. At the request of the publisher, the discussion on hypnosis has been edited in a similar manner.

The participants in the discussion on Hypnosis in Anesthesiology had agreed, prior to the meeting, on a list of questions to be debated, and Dr. STOKVIS' introductory statement on the nature of hypnosis was circulated among them in appropriate translations in order to give the debate a starting point.

It had also been agreed that no formal papers should be read after this introduction, and that the participants should use at will the German, English or French language. Following each contribution it was the chairman's task to give a brief summary in the two other languages. Discussion was therefore somewhat slowed down and occasionally rendered difficult by misunderstandings or the omission of details.

Drs. GUÉGUEN, MOSCONI, and VÖLGYESI, who were not able to attend, had sent written contributions which the chairman presented briefly during the discussion.

The present text has been worked out of the tape recording of the discussion and the chairman's correspondence with the panelists some time after the meeting. Whenever the original contributions were in French or German, the English translation has been the chairman's.

130, rue de la Pompe   JEAN LASSNER
Paris XVI, France

Contents

Introduction 1

The nature of hypnosis 2

Hypnosis and the doctor-patient relationship in
anesthesiology 5

The indications for hypnosis in anesthesiology 9

The induction of hypnosis 10

Hypnosis in pediatric anesthesia 13

Drugs and hypnosis 14

Neurophysiological effects of hypnosis 17

Clinical aspects of hypnoanesthesia 20
    A. Surgery 20
    B. Obstetrics 21
    C. Hypnosis and the neuro-endocrine response . . . 24
    D. Hypnosis in emergency operations 26
    E. Hypnosis in E.N.T. surgery 32
    F. Hypnosis for hypothermia 34
    G. Hypnosis in dental surgery 35

Difficulties and dangers 37

Conclusion 50

HYPNOSIS IN ANESTHESIOLOGY

AN INTERNATIONAL SYMPOSIUM

HELD AT THE FIRST EUROPEAN CONGRESS OF ANESTHESIOLOGY
OF THE
WORLD FEDERATION OF SOCIETIES OF ANESTHESIOLOGISTS

VIENNA / AUSTRIA, SEPTEMBER 5, 1962

CHAIRMAN AND EDITOR

JEAN LASSNER, M. D.
PARIS, FRANCE

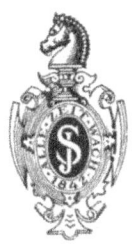

SPRINGER-VERLAG
BERLIN · GÖTTINGEN · HEIDELBERG
1964

All rights, especially that of translation into foreign languages, reserved.
It is also forbidden to reproduce this book, either whole or in part, by photomechanical means
(photostat, microfilm and/or microcard) or by other procedure without written permission from
Springer-Verlag

ISBN-13:978-3-540-03166-6   e-ISBN-13:978-3-642-46003-6
DOI:10.1007/978-3-642-46003-6

© by Springer-Verlag OHG Berlin · Göttingen · Heidelberg 1964

Library of Congress Catalog Card Number 64—20590

The reproduction of general descriptive names, trade names, trade marks, etc. in this
publication, even when there is no special identification mark, is not to be taken as a
sign that such names, as understood by the Trade Marks and Merchandise Marks Law,
may accordingly be freely used by anyone.

Printed by Konrad Triltsch, Graphischer Großbetrieb, Würzburg
Titel-Nr. 1231

Participants

JOVAN ANTITCH   English
38 Dosilejeva St., Belgrade, Yugoslavia

BASIL FINER   English
Murargatan 30 D, Uppsala, Sweden

JEAN GUÉGUEN   French
10, rue Raynouard, Paris 16, France

LAWRENCE GOLDIE   English
Hammersmith Hospital, Du Cane Road,
Shepherds Bush, London W. 12, England

MILTON J. MARMER   English
507 North Arden Drive,
Beverly Hills, California, U. S. A.

GIAMPIERO MOSCONI   French
Via Pacini 37, Milan, Italy

BERNARD B. RAGINSKY   English
376 Redfern Avenue, Montreal, Quebec, Canada

OTTO SCHMID-SCHMIDSFELDEN   German
Theodor-Körner-Straße 65, Graz, Austria

GUNTHER SEMELKA   German
Hôpital Général, St. Boniface, Manitoba, Canada

RUDOLF STERN   German
Palazzo "La Ginevrina," Lugano, Switzerland

BERTHOLD STOKVIS *   German
c/o Jelgersma-Kliniek, Oegstgeest, Holland

---

* Dr. STOKVIS died suddenly on September 8th, 1963.

TAMÁS VÁNDOR   German
Institut für Anaesthesiologie der Universität,
Mainz, Germany

FERENC VÖLGYESI   German
Bajcsy-Zsilinszky Ut 23, Budapest, Hungary

J. WILLIAM WOODWARD   English
50 Broadway North, Walsall, Staffordshire
England

MARTIN ZWICKER   German
Stadtkrankenhaus, Soest, Germany

Introduction

Chairman: When the executive committee of this First European Congress of Anesthesiology decided to schedule a panel discussion on hypnosis it must have been under the influence of forces operative nowhere else but in this city of Vienna. As far as I am aware, this topic has never before been on the agenda of a meeting of anesthetists. At the request of the executive committee, it became my task to invite participants and structure the debate of this panel. Under these circumstances, it seems appropriate that I should make an initial statement of intent.

Hypnosis has been a highly controversial subject ever since it made its entrance into modern medicine at the end of the 18th century in this city. The esteem in which it was held as a therapeutic tool and the prevailing opinion concerning its practice have known successively great peaks and depressions. There has been a renewed interest in hypnosis in the English-speaking countries during the last few years. At the same time, a psychological method for pain relief during childbirth, developed in Russia as an offspring of hypnotic analgesia, has been widely acclaimed in France and Italy. Here and there, anesthetists have become interested in this matter, but their experiences are few and isolated. Obviously, there is a tremendous gap between the usual field of activity anesthetists are accustomed to the world over and hypnosis.

Our first aim has therefore been to assume an approach to the subject under discussion. At the same time, a common basis was to be found for our debate. Since there are various and opposing views on hypnosis, this latter endeavour seemed to be of prime importance in order to avoid spurious arguments. It is our privilege to have among the members of this panel Dr. B. Stokvis, whose wide knowledge in this field is universally esteemed. He has been good enough to prepare a statement on the nature of hypnosis on which we have agreed to base our discussion.

The first topic to be debated will then be the question of how the use of hypnosis by an anesthetist will influence his way of practising our speciality and, more specifically, how this will modify the patient-doctor relationship in this field.

Nobody would use any particular form of therapy in every case. So this brings up the question of when to use hypnosis. Once agreed on how to determine when hypnosis would be indicated, another problem arises. It is well known that one cannot induce hypnosis in everyone. To choose appropriate cases comes therefore to mean also such cases where hypnosis may succeed. Eventually this will lead to the question of how to ensure success in a given case. This will bring up the matter of induction methods and the ability of the anesthetist to practise hypnosis.

Here I would like to add a word to prevent erroneous expectations. It is not our purpose to teach such methods here.

We will then come to speak of hypnosis in its application to the various fields of surgery, obstetrics and dentistry. Several motion pictures will be shown illustrating these possibilities.

Afterwards we will discuss the difficulties and resistances encountered when using hypnosis, and finally the dangers and complications possibly resulting from its use.

I am quite aware that this is a very ambitious programme for a rather short meeting. Many questions will have to be summarily treated for reasons of time. So let us begin by asking Dr. STOKVIS for his conception of the nature of hypnosis.

The nature of hypnosis

Stokvis: Hypnosis can be understood only from a psychosomatic point of view. It encompasses all the manifestations of the human being and is induced through affective influences which appear in the individual's experience and in his body. It is therefore part of the emotional life.

Neither the psychological nor the physiological theories of hypnosis are appropriate. Hypnosis is an alteration of the psychosomatic unity produced by affective resonance. It entails a modification of consciousness, frequently giving the hypnotized person the appearance of being asleep. How consciousness is modified depends mainly on autosuggestive influences. Each person produces his own type of hypnosis. There is no one sign constantly present in hypnotized people. That is probably why BABINSKY considered hypnosis a fraud. Studies on how hypnosis is experienced have shown that it entails a certain regression in personality structure as well as in bodily functions. This regression may reactivate emotional reactions of the Oedipus situation. Hypnosis is an archaic state which can be accompanied by modifications in the autonomic and endocrine functions, probably induced by the hypothalamus.

Scientific approach can be made to hypnosis through: 1) experimental medico-psychological study; 2) psychodiagnostic methods; 3) studies in clinical psychology; 4) studies in physio-psychology.

Our medico-psychological studies have been conducted along phenomenological and psychoanalytic lines. The world of the hypnotized seems to be like the world of a child whom an adult has taken by the hand. Occasionally the world of the hypnotized seems to be quite similar to the one experienced by a hysteric. Our psychoanalytical studies have demonstrated that the behaviour of the hypnotized depends not only on his constitution and autosuggestive imagination but is determined also by the doctor-patient relationship. The latter constitutes a transference relationship. Both positive and negative effects can be demonstrated. The form and the effects taken by hypnosis are therefore determined to a great extent by the patient's infantile conditionment. The operator can constitute for the patient a father as well as a mother image, for in deep hypnosis the Oedipus situation, or even a fear of castration, can be reactivated. The patient's behaviour is also determined by the urge to pleasurable self-abandonment. These hetero- or homo-erotic feelings help the hypnotized to identify himself with the operator and to introject the latter's orders. Each patient attributes some magic capacities to the physician, and through identification he takes part in the magic power. That is how the regression into the magic world is achieved, and that is why such extensive effects can be obtained through suggestion in hypnosis. In psychoanalytical terminology, it is through the hypnotizer's penis that the hypnotized achieves great power.

A word about our psychodiagnostic studies. A battery of tests systematically performed have shown regressive phenomena affecting, in hypnosis, the whole personality: modifications have been shown to affect the intelligence, motor expression, affectivity, character and temperament. Our graphological studies have shown that reality testing is lost very rarely; it is an essential feature of hypnosis that the suggested situation is actively experienced while a more or less clear notion of reality is maintained. This means that the hypnotized is frequently aware that he is playing a role. This induces disagreeable feelings in the observer.

As reported in our clinical-psychological studies, there is no specific sign of hypnosis to be observed in the hypnotized. This holds true also for catalepsy, which can be missing even in deep hypnosis. Theoretically, every modification induced by emotions could be produced through hypnosis. In fact, resistances frequently come into play.

We have been able to complete our physio-psychological studies these last years with the use of an electronic polygraph. We have been able to show that through hypnotic suggestion every physiological function can be modified. Obviously suggestibility is increased in hypnosis. This does not mean that hypnosis can be induced only in suggestible persons.

Chairman: Dr. STOKVIS' introduction was circulated among the members of this panel prior to the present meeting. Several dissenting opinions have been voiced, as was to be expected. Supporters of one or the other of the theories of hypnosis, be it the naturalistic approach with its two main variants, the Pavlovian and the behaviouristic, or the anthropological approach, have contested some of the statements just made. The psychoanalytical interpretations derived from FERENCZI's work have been strongly criticized. But in order to reach the real subject matter of today's meeting, we have agreed nevertheless not to open a discussion on theory.

To modify emotions and physiological function, or to prevent the latter's deterioration, is a matter of great interest to anesthetists. Let us take this as a starting point for a discussion of the first question which comes up: what could the role of hypnosis be in anesthesia, and how does its practice affect the relationship between the anesthetist and his patient? May I ask Dr. STOKVIS to continue.

Hypnosis and the doctor-patient relationship in anesthesiology

Stokvis: Hypnosis has been used in anesthesiology to achieve pre-operative sedation. It has occasionally been used as the sole means of achieving anesthesia, or it has been combined with chemical anesthesia. It has been shown to facilitate post-operative recovery. Hypnosis can abolish sensitivity and reduce or eliminate the anxiety frequently linked to the experience of pain. This effect has been compared to the one obtained by prefrontal leucotomy. The dissociation of pain experience from suffering can also be of help in chronic pain conditions.

In anesthesiology hypnosis is therefore mainly useful to achieve psychosomatic changes.

Whether hypnosis should be used depends on the personality of the patient, the personality of the physician, the symptoms present, and on the social and economic set-up. The symptoms should not be considered alone. In hypnosis, as in other forms of psychotherapy, it is not so much the method of treatment as the doctor who helps the patient.

There are many cases in anesthesiology where hypnosis is unnecessary, and some where it should not be used. When the preliminary interview leads to suppose that hypnosis might produce unpleasant effects by way of autosuggestion, one should proceed with great caution. If the patient refuses hypnosis, one should certainly not use it. One should probably abstain also when the interview reveals a hysterical personality. In impending psychosis, hypnosis is to be avoided except in involutional depression.

Chairman: While for a long time interest among anesthetists has been focussed primarily on pharmacology and physiology, there have been many contributions in recent years aiming at a better understanding of the patient's psychological situation. Still, there is a long way from the position of a critical observer to the assumption of an articulate psychotherapeutic management. The latter no doubt requires a major change in the actual practice, at least as far as the relationship between the anesthetist and his patient is concerned. I would like to ask Dr. RAGINSKY to give us his opinion in this matter.

Raginsky: Inter-personal relationships in hypnosis are much deeper and more meaningful than at non-hypnotic levels. In other words, any mishandling of the normal relationship with a patient is greatly magnified when it occurs in connection with a hypnotized patient. As compared to chemo-anesthesia, hypnosis, whether it be used to achieve a state of painlessness or any other hypnotic effect, implies a much greater involvement of both patient and doctor. It also usually requires more time from the latter. Aside from technical skill in the use of hypnosis, he must also have a keen awareness of the patient's emotional needs. He must be able to recognize whether a particular patient should have a passive induction or an authoritarian one. Thus the physician must be flexible and resourceful in meeting the patient's requirements if the subsequent patient-physician relationship is to remain constructive.

Nothing should be told the patient in the hypnotic state that the doctor would not tell him in the waking state. If sufficient care is taken in the course of induction to obtain the patient's cooperation, he will come out of the experience with a somewhat stronger ego than before. Alternatively, if the patient has been bullied into submission, there may be posthypnotic hostility. To maintain a good patient-physician relationship, it is essential not to disturb a patient's image of himself.

The patient-physician relationship following hypnoanesthesia is usually better than in most other hypnotic situations. This is so because the objectives are simple and direct, and do not usually interfere with the patient's emotional equilibrium.

Chairman: It will be of interest to hear how the use of hypnosis has affected the anesthetist's daily routine.

Semelka: At least in North America, the relationship between the anesthetist and the patient is often superficial. The anesthetist is considered as a rather impersonal agent, an efficient technician, not a person.

By the act of inducing hypnosis, the anesthetist demonstrates his special interest in the patient, who in turn shows that he accepts him by going into hypnosis. Therefore hypnosis adds a new dimension to the patient-anesthetist relationship, deepening their mutual appreciation. To what degree depends on the purpose of the hypnosis and the circumstances under which it is administered. Hypnoid suggestions often go unnoticed when used to make the induction of anesthesia by injection or inhalation more acceptable. Group hypnosis, as in maternity classes, makes a fairly deep impression on the patients. Hypnosis used in the treatment of pain unrelieved by other means or in terminal disease states knits a close tie between the anesthetist and his patient.

Völgyesi: Since I started my private hypnotherapeutic practice in 1918, I have been called upon a great number of times by colleagues in the surgical field for various reasons. Certain patients show extreme anxiety, and in this case many surgeons feel that the operation is fraught with danger. In this circumstance, as well as with highly neurotic patients who cope badly with the stress of hospitalization and the sickness itself, hypnosis offers a tremendous help. On the other hand, there are a good number of patients with severe heart disease or other conditions that make general anesthesia difficult or dangerous, some also have allergies or sensitivities to various drugs. Hypnoanesthesia is then the method of choice. I have been able to demonstrate this very vividly at a meeting, held in Budapest on July 1, 1922, of the Hungarian society of dentists. The patient, a dentist himself, had phobic fear of dental care, he was suffering from advanced rheumatic heart disease, and was allergic to novocaine. As a result, his denture had been severely neglected. Under hypnosis, three teeth were extracted at the meeting without any reaction on the part of the patient.

Chairman: Hypnosis certainly increases the therapeutic possibilities of the anesthetist. It therefore heightens, so to speak, his professional status, and modifies his relations with both patients and other doctors. It is our privilege to have among us a surgeon who has also been practising anesthesia and hypnosis.

To terminate our discussion of this point I would like to ask Professor ZWICKER to give us his opinion on the relationship between anesthetist and patient when hypnosis is used.

Zwicker: The development of highly technical means of investigation and of operative techniques of increasing complexity have led to a practice of surgery in which the personal contact between the patient and the surgeon has been very much reduced. The great work load in hospitals also explains why surgeons are chronically short of time. These changed conditions have not modified the patient's need for assistance in the stress-filled situation created by the impending operation. We can only to a certain extent replace confidence in the individual surgeon by belief in surgery anonymously practised. The present conditions in surgical hospitals therefore increase the need for psychotherapy. It does not matter whether this psychotherapy is given by the surgeon or the anesthetist, but the latter seems to be in a better position to accomplish it.

The central problem of this therapy should be, in my opinion, the pre-operative fear of the patient, which stems from uncertainty about the outcome of illness and operation, and from the feeling of being abandoned. The pre-operative visit of the anesthetist offers a possibility to help the patient by a detailed discussion of these matters. Should this be insufficient, suggestions in the waking state or hypnosis can be very useful psychotherapeutic tools. In this way, the first steps are taken to prepare the patient actively for the post-operative recovery. Thanks to hypnosis, this period can become much more pleasant, and many of its features positively influenced—postanesthetic vomiting, micturition, bowel movements and appetite and, last but not least, post-operative pain.

I have been able to perform a number of operations under hypnosis, or under hypnosis combined with local anesthesia. The main value of hypnotic analgesia is to demonstrate the effectiveness of hypnosis through the relief of pain. In the modern practice of anesthesia there will seldom if ever be a need of hypnosis to achieve anesthesia. No doubt the chemical methods are simpler and require much less time. But for the pre- and post-operative treatment, psychotherapeutic methods are undoubtedly superior to the chemical ones.

Chairman: It seems that we agree on the added possibilities given the anesthetist by including psychotherapy and hypnosis in his professional radius. Obviously this does not mean that every patient undergoing surgery or anesthesia needs psychotherapy or hypnosis. This brings up the question of when to use hypnosis.

The indications for hypnosis in anesthesiology

Marmer: The choice of a suitable case is patient-determined, as is everything else in hypnosis. In order to know when and when not to use hypnosis, the patient must be seen by the anesthesiologist pre-operatively. If the patient appears to be relaxed and easy-going, without façade, confident and emotionally stable, if the patient already has the proper "psychological set" for the anticipated surgery and anesthesia, and if the patient offers physiological evidence of the validity of this impression, such as a warm, dry skin, a normal, regular pulse rate, and a normal blood pressure, then this patient should be left alone with reference to hypnosis. The anesthesiologist should have a pleasant visit with such a patient and not upset him in any way.

On the other hand, if the patient appears to be apprehensive and agitated, and asks a thousand and one questions, relevant and irrelevant, he needs more attention. When the agitation is accompanied by a cold, clammy skin, tachycardia and elevated blood pressure, occasionally even hyperventilation, you have all the corroborative evidence of a nervous, fearful, tense patient. This patient needs hypnosis, especially if he tells you, "Doctor, I am afraid I am going to die." Do not ever shrug such a statement off. Do not ever take it as a joke. Such patients may die, and need all the emotional support you are capable of giving them.

When I first started experimenting with hypnosis, I used it in every case. I had not yet developed any criteria for its use. As I gained more experience, I developed not only personal confidence, but a sixth sense which enabled me to actually choose the right patients for the use of hypnosis. There are situations where the use of hypnosis becomes more mandatory, such as in traumatic procedures where the patient has a full stomach and in very poor risk patients. Recently I was called upon to attempt hypnosis on a child who was burned very severely in an accident. The accident had taken place one month prior to my seeing the patient. I attempted hypnosis but it was of no avail. This was like closing the barn door after the horse had been stolen. In order to use hypnosis successfully in these cases, it must be used from the very beginning of therapy.

Chairman: As Dr. MARMER just pointed out, once hypnosis has been deemed indicated, attempts to achieve it can succeed or fail. In the case of the burned child, Dr. MARMER felt that the failure was due to the fact that the child had lost confidence in doctors. This shows that the patient's situation influences the outcome of the attempt, but could also be interpreted to mean that the method of induction was not appropriate for the given case. Instead of looking for subjects who are easily hypnotized, as is the case in experimental hypnosis, the object of medical hypnosis is to succeed in inducing it in a given patient. It seems therefore appropriate that we now discuss the methods of induction available to the anesthetist.

The induction of hypnosis

Stokvis: Whatever technique of induction is to be used, it has to be adapted to the individual patient. This means first of all that the patient must be prepared in a preliminary interview. At the same time the interview is needed to obtain information about the patient. The patient's cooperation must be ensured, whether we choose to inform him or not that hypnosis will be used.

As in other fields of medical practice, the physician may feel more at ease with certain techniques than with others. To adapt himself to the patient's needs he has to be proficient with several. Nevertheless, success is likely to be achieved most often with the doctor's preferred method. Our own preference consists in having the patient look fixedly at a card showing two contrasting colours. This method was first described by MAX LEVY-SUHL in 1908. While the patient looks at the grey interval between the two coloured strips, one yellow, the other blue, the appropriate suggestions are given to the effect that the complementary colours will appear in the grey interval. We find this method rapid in execution, certain in effect, and easily accepted by the patient.

Induction by verbal suggestion alone, which is the most frequently used procedure today, seems to have a greater failure rate than its combination with eye fixation. Instead of using our colour card for this purpose, any brilliant object may be used. A well-known variant of the fixation method consists in having the patient stare into the doctor's eyes. The latter technique is very tiring for the doctor and may occasionally have an erotizing effect. It is therefore to be reserved for exceptional circumstances. Besides this optical stimulus, other sensory stimuli can be used. Only those concerning touch are of practical importance, particularly a rhythmical soft stroking, the so-called passes used by MESMER. Here again the erotizing effect is obvious.

The use of barbiturates or other drugs to facilitate induction is unwarranted and amounts to admitting a fear of failure on the part of the practitioner.

It is of interest to note that modern literature on hypnosis has added nothing essential to the techniques already indicated by the pioneers.

Marmer: Methods of induction of hypnosis depend upon the personality of the hypnotist and his evaluation of the patient. The most universal method, but one which takes the most time, is any variation on the technique of "Progressive Relaxation."

Find the technique that suits your personality best. The more subtle the approach and the less dramatic it is, the more successful will be the result. Your voice should convey a sense of assurance and confidence. In essence, there should never be an aura of mystery or any ceremoniousness about the procedure. The less ritualistic and the more straightforward the hypnotic technique, the better. Suggestions should be repeated as one progresses through the muscular system of the body, constantly suggesting relaxation, ease, peace of mind, drowsiness and sleepiness.

Another technique which is successful in the hands of many practitioners is the phenomenon of levitation. This sometimes gives the patient an opportunity to "play act" and is often difficult to evaluate as to validity of hypnotic depth. Other techniques which I have used have been the stethoscope method, and the use of a respiration simulator. The stethoscope method begins with the examination of the patient's chest, getting the patient to breathe deeply, in and out, in and out, and progressively extending the suggestions to include the sensation of drowsiness and sleepiness. This has the unique benefit of beginning with what the patient expects and then suggesting the unexpected. It is very valid because of the average person's familiarity with the stethoscope.

Very recently, a small machine which produces sounds simulating respiration has been marketed in the United States, with the idea of training pulmonary emphysema patients and other pulmonary cripples to breathe more deeply and to regulate the rate of respiration by following the sounds of the Respiratory Simulator. I have been able to use this machine in several instances to induce hypnosis. This is merely an extension of the experiments conducted by Kubie and Margolin on the use of respiratory sounds as a hypnogogic stimulus. I must admit that no one else in my hospital who tried it was able to achieve the same success. There is no question about the fact that the personality and skill of the individual hypnotist, rather than any specialized technique, plays the major role in induction.

For the achievement of analgesia and anesthesia, the most successful technique has been that of "glove anesthesia." Methods of deepening anesthesia are very variable and depend primarily on the individual.

Chairman: I quite agree with Dr. Marmer on the importance of choosing an approach that fits into the framework of the anesthetist's usual pre-operative visit. It is for this reason that I have been using for some time elements of the routine neurological examination as means of hypnotic induction. This is an elaboration of the procedure recommended by Dr. Ainslie Meares, who has demonstrated the significance of the various responses of patients to the examination of the patellar reflex.

I must say that I am less hesitant than Dr. Stokvis to use the effects of touch. In certain circumstances, massage can be an excellent method of induction—in the case of a patient complaining of post-operative muscular pain, for example. We do not avoid a rectal or vaginal examination in clinical practice when indicated, although we all know their important psychological implications. As to the use of gadgets to facilitate induction, they are mainly helpful to give the doctor assurance or to increase his prestige with the patient. Maybe we can devote a few more minutes to special problems of induction: first of all, hypnosis with children; secondly, the combined use of hypnosis and drugs.

Hypnosis in pediatric anesthesia

Goldie: Children are the easiest subjects for hypnosis when there is an operation in the offing and an anesthetic to be given. The anxiety of the child is proportional to his suggestibility, and the most anxious child will often respond best. The terror-stricken child whose fears seriously hinder the institution of treatment will benefit by hypnosis unless there is time to cope with his fears in some other way.

It is easy with this type of patient to produce an effect by simple suggestion. But this suggestion should never follow the pattern of a ritual. If something goes wrong in the ritualistic procedure, the result will be psychological chaos that is damaging to the patient and makes future psychological handling difficult. What is needed is the application of rational psychological insight and not adherence to any specific hypnotic technique, otherwise hypnosis could easily become a magic means to dispel the doctor's and the patient's fears.

An anesthetist using hypnosis without a knowledge of psychology would be unable to learn from his mistakes when something goes wrong.

The reason for not using hypnosis as a ritual with children lies in the fact that it is our duty to aid the child and not to retard its process of maturation. We have to promote trust in adults as rational people and contradict unbridled fantasy by our behaviour, fostering contact with reality. This rule will occasionally result in the rejection of hypnosis so as to give the child an opportunity to cope with the situation without extra help. In this way the anesthetist can contribute to the development of a strong ego and conscience.

Pain and anxiety are inevitable in children as in adults. Our aim is to contradict fantasy by consistent behaviour and truthful answers to questions. We should even encourage questions, thereby showing that the doctor is not insecure. However great anxieties may be despite the explanations given, the child will then find the truth confirmed and frightening fantasies contradicted. In this way, sufficient strength will be developed to stand pain and depression with courage. As an outcome the child will eventually react with reason and not avoid issues. Anesthetists are present on unique occasions in a child's life and should not be disturbed by their patients' anxieties to the point of resorting too easily to procedures such as hypnosis.

Marmer: I agree with Dr. GOLDIE's statement that it is easy to induce hypnosis in children. I also share his view that we should not adhere to a ritual in inducing it. I find it quite practical to have children simply imagine they are looking at a television screen after having found out about their favourite programme. It is then suggested that they visualize a scene ending in somebody going to sleep, and finally the suggestions are switched to have them relax in the same way.

I disagree with Dr. GOLDIE's interpretation of hypnosis as an escape mechanism. I feel it should be considered as a means of fostering control in a given situation; it can then be incorporated by the child in his maturation process as a form of achievement.

Chairman: Dr. GOLDIE's remarks show again how closely the indication of hypnosis and induction methods are related. Dr. STOKVIS has expressed opposition to the use of drugs to facilitate induction. I would now like to hear Dr. WOODWARD on this very controversial subject.

Drugs and hypnosis

Woodward: I would rather comment on the combined use of drugs and hypnosis. It has been noted for a long time that the efficiency of various local and general anesthetic agents can be increased by hypnosis. It has also been said that the use of drugs facilitates induction of the hypnotic state. In our opinion, drugs like most of the phenothiazine derivatives which act on the reticular system in the brain stem, depressing the central activating system, make the patient less apprehensive. These same drugs also raise the pain threshold. They may facilitate hypnosis as well, and we may postulate that the reticular system is involved in the production of a trance state.

We are satisfied when we can reduce the amount of anesthetic or analgesic drugs employed by raising the pain threshold through hypnosis. There is no reason why the anesthetic agent should not be used to facilitate hypnotic induction. Induction of hypnosis may sometimes proceed pari-passu with induction of anesthesia by a mixture of 80% nitrous oxide and 20% oxygen, or by a slow intravenous injection of 2.5% thiopentone. The combination of nitrous oxide-oxygen inhalation and hypnosis will produce a mental state in which suggestions are readily accepted by the patient. The patient is usually conscious when teeth are extracted by this method. He may remember the extraction, but will not protest. He may be aware of what is going on, but will not be disturbed and will feel no pain. It may be usefully mentioned that alcohol is one of the oldest drugs used in the relief of pain and that it may also facilitate hypnotic induction.

Since reduced amounts of analgesic drugs become sufficient when used in combination with hypnosis, this combination should be resorted to whenever the depressant effects of a larger dose of these drugs is to be avoided. This is obviously the case after any operation where early full control of the air passages is essential, like tonsillectomies and dental extractions.

Chairman: The conflict of opinion between Dr. STOKVIS and Dr. WOODWARD apparently stems from the difference in purpose. In a psychotherapeutic setting, which is usually the case with Dr. STOKVIS, the achievement of hypnosis becomes a goal in itself for both the patient and the therapist. To facilitate induction by drugs may easily be construed as depriving the achievement of part of its value. We are faced here with the question of the interaction of psychopharmacology and psychotherapy.

Dr. WOODWARD's mention of nitrous oxide analgesia reminds us of the earliest descriptions of this gas's effects. During a lecture demonstration given by GARDENER Q. COLTON on December 10, 1844, in Hartford, Connecticut, a man named Sam Cooley, who had inhaled nitrous oxide, stumbled while getting up and cut his shin open without showing any sign of pain. It was by observing this event that HORACE WELLS came to think of nitrous oxide inhalation as a means of making surgery painless even without suggestion. By applying anesthetic agents in a suitable way, analgesia without loss of consciousness can certainly be achieved. The short inhalation of ether was called "*Rausch*" by German authors at the end of the last century. This means a short-lived drunkenness during which brief surgical procedure can be performed. SUDEK in 1901, and SCHMIDT some twenty-five years later, showed how this analgesic state could be prolonged. In 1955 ARTUSIO again drew attention to ether analgesia.

To come back to nitrous oxide and hypnosis, Dr. RAGINSKY published in 1937, I believe, a very interesting study showing how its effects depended on the mental state of the patient. Perhaps we could ask him to comment on this matter.

Raginsky: The object of our study at that time can certainly be related to Dr. WOODWARD's findings. Dental patients were purposely made anxious by disturbing behaviour on the part of the dentist and his assistants. These anxious patients could not be anesthetized by nitrous oxide without increasing the percentage so as to create anoxia. In patients put at ease, 80% or less of nitrous oxide gave satisfactory results.

Chairman: We will discuss later the use of nitrous oxide in dental surgery. At the present time I would like to draw a parallel between the behaviour of Dr. RAGINSKY's dental patients and the struggling and agitation one can observe in certain surgical patients when they emerge from an anesthetic. Such agitation is more frequent in patients who are heavy drinkers, drug addicts, or very tense, nervous individuals. These facts may be interpreted along the following lines: the patient stays quiet as long as he is fully unconscious or fully relieved of pain. When pain is experienced while consciousness is still clouded, agitation may occur. Patients accustomed to inhibiting drugs or inclined to a state of excessive vigilance will become partially conscious more rapidly than others.

One is then offered the not very attractive choice of unduly increasing the dosage of analgesics or of retarding the full recovery from the anesthetic by drugs like the ataractics. In our experience hypnosis can be induced rather easily in this situation as long as no restraint is imposed on the patient's muscular activities. The critical phase can be easily overcome in this way.

The combined actions of drugs and hypnosis as outlined in Dr. WOODWARD's and Dr. RAGINSKY's remarks bring up the question of the neurophysiology involved. Before discussing the use of hypnosis in the various surgical fields, I would therefore like to ask Dr. FINER to give us a short synopsis of his experimental findings in this field.

Neurophysiological effects of hypnosis

Finer: Using electromyography, with needles inserted into the vastus medialis, we have studied the withdrawal reflex produced by applying painful electrical stimuli to the skin on the anterior and posterior surface of the lower leg. Two types of stimuli were used: short ones of 20 to 40 msec., resulting in a spinal withdrawal reflex of a latency of 60 to 80 msec.; and long stimuli of 200 msec. where the stimulus is interrupted by the withdrawal movement itself, resulting in a spinal reflex with a latency of 60 to 80 msec. and a later reflex with a latency of 120 msec. probably conditioned in nature. The spinal reflex is relatively stable and unadaptable. It increases with apprehension, spontaneous or suggested, and decreases with monotony, spontaneous or suggested. It is sometimes increased during hypnotic hyperalgesia and sometimes decreased during hypnotic analgesia. The "conditioned" reflex is relatively unstable and adaptable. It always produces a response that is appropriate to the total situation. It increases with apprehension, spontaneous or suggested, and decreases with monotony, spontaneous or suggested. It can be taught to change to a reflex inhibition if the situation is appropriate, sometimes opposing the spinal reflex. It is markedly increased by hypnotic hyperalgesia and decreased by hypnotic analgesia. During hypnotic analgesia of the foot, the plantar reflex usually decreases or disappears. This change can be assessed or recorded as an objective test for the hypnotic state.

Stokvis: I wonder whether these experiments conclusively show that the spinal reflex arc is modified through hypnosis. Dr. WOODWARD has suggested that we should look to the reticular formation in the mid-brain as the neurophysiological substratum of hypnosis. Blocking of afferent impulses certainly occurs, as has been shown by electroencephalographic studies.

Chairman: Thirty years ago, BASS attempted to demonstrate the difference between hypnosis and sleep by showing that the patellar reflex is present in hypnosis whereas it disappears during sleep. Dr. FINER wants to demonstrate the difference between the waking state and hypnosis through the possibility of abolishing in hypnosis the plantar withdrawal reflex induced by strong electrical stimulation. Many of you are probably familiar with the various papers published recently by BARBER, who tries to demonstrate the opposite. He seems to want to negate hypnosis by showing that whatever has been observed in people under hypnosis can also be done without a formal hypnotic induction. If we keep in mind Dr. GOLDIE's statement about avoiding a ritual, one may wonder whether some of BARBER's subjects did not actually achieve hypnosis without a formal induction. If so, his experiments mainly showed that hypnosis can occur spontaneously or be induced without a ritual. But I should like to ask Dr. FINER whether he has done experiments to find out if one can prevent the withdrawal reflex at will or only when strongly ordered to do so.

Finer: When testing for hypnotic analgesia by pricking a patient's skin with a needle, one certainly leaves it to the subject to decide whether or not to demonstrate pain by gestures or words. Nearly everybody could abstain from such demonstrations if he wanted to. I don't feel that a similar choice is offered in the case of strong electrical stimulation of the foot.

Perhaps it would be appropriate to mention here another study which we have conducted. We have elicited nystagmus by rotatory and caloric vestibular stimuli and recorded it by electronystagmography. Hypnosis and suggestion of increased rotation increased the nystagmus response, while hypnosis and suggestion of decreased rotation decreased the nystagmus response. Hypnosis without suggestion or vestibular stimulation produced responses similar to those that occur during "slow cerebration," that is, deep unconsciousness or barbiturate intoxication.

Since we are now going to discuss clinical matters, I would like to relate our attempts to improve lung function after cholecystectomy in women by training in hypnotic analgesia before the operation. Lung function was assessed by $FEV_{1.0}$, and peak expiratory flow on the day before the operation and every day for four days after the operation. However, no difference in performance could be noted between those trained in hypnosis and controls. Subjectively, many of the hypnotic subjects said that they felt less pain. Further experiments are in progress.

Raginsky: I am happy to hear that you are continuing your experiments and are not ready to draw conclusions from these findings. There are great differences in the results achieved by using hypnosis, depending on the time and effort available for the individual patient, the experience of the practitioner, and the degree of sophistication in the use of hypnosis. Instead of suggesting analgesia to obtain better lung function, various imagined settings requiring heavy breathing might have been substituted.

Chairman: May I draw attention to Dr. FINER's finding of a different response according to whether hypnosis with or without suggestions of increased or decreased rotation was used in his nystagmus experiments. Since the induction of hypnosis most of the time bears some similarity to falling asleep, suggestions of drowsiness or sleep are often given. Feelings of bodily relaxation may evoke associations implying sleep even without any suggestions of this type being formulated. It is therefore difficult to ascertain whether the described state of "slow cerebration" is characteristic of hypnosis per se or only when it is induced in a certain way. The matter is of great theoretic interest, since many therapists have expressed the opinion that "hypnosis per se" is capable of producing powerful effects, while others consider it only a vehicle for treatment, much in the way one may use a syringe to inject any drug deemed useful.

But perhaps we could start the discussion of clinical aspects by considering the unusual but very spectacular use of hypnosis as sole means to achieve anesthesia, or rather analgesia.

Clinical aspects of hypnoanesthesia

A) Surgery

Marmer: It is only in isolated and rare instances that hypnosis can be used to perform painlessly any surgical procedure. Its possibilities are limited in the case of surgical interventions requiring profound muscular relaxation. Greater opportunity in using hypnosis alone is afforded to the anesthetist in minor surgical procedures, emergencies, simple operations with children, and in those instances where the patient is to go home shortly after the operation is performed.

Where muscular relaxation is provided for by nature, as with cesarean section or cesarean hysterectomy, the procedures can be carried out under hypnoanesthesia without much difficulty and with greater frequency. Hypnoanalgesia and hypnoanesthesia are also very valid techniques for pulmonary and cardiac surgery. Only one requirement of anesthesia in thoracic surgery cannot be achieved by hypnosis, and that is the control of respiration in order to provide the surgeon with an absolutely quiet operative field. When this becomes compulsory, it is necessary to administer small doses of succinylcholine. Respiration is then assisted or controlled according to the completeness of the chemical apnoea which results. Endotracheal intubation can be performed under hypnosis but requires greater dexterity because it is not as easily performed as with a completely chemically anesthetized and relaxed patient.

The use of hypnosis as a means of anesthesia requires the surgeon's as well as the patient's cooperation. Consequently, I use it with certain surgeons only, namely those who have confidence in me as a hypnotist, those who do not talk too much during surgery, and those who handle tissues gently and with dexterity.

Chairman: It is well to remember that the possibility of performing surgery painlessly in patients under hypnosis was used long before the discovery of chemical anesthesia. CLOQUET performed a mammectomy in Paris in 1829 on a mesmerized patient. But the shortcomings of this method are also well known. It certainly cannot compete with chemo-anesthesia in a modern surgical hospital. I think no one familiar with hypnosis could conceive of such a competition, nor judge hypnosis by its results.

One of the most fruitful fields for the application of hypnosis seems to have been its use to alleviate the pains of childbirth. I would like to ask Drs. MOSCONI and GUÉGUEN to comment on this.

B) Obstetrics

Mosconi: Hypnosis has been used in obstetrics on and off for a century and a half. Interest in its use has increased recently in Italy as a means of psychological preparation aiming less at abolishing pain than at achieving the active participation of the woman in labour. Frequently analgesia is achieved by this means alone. If we agree to READ's trilogy of fear, tension and pain, we will find in hypnosis the most efficient means to prevent pain during the confinement. In fact, confidence, relaxation and a tranquil mind achieved through its use will be of great help during pregnancy also. In cooperation with different obstetricians we have been conducting preparatory sessions both with individual patients and with groups since 1957. Our results have been most gratifying. The economy of time in preparing groups of patients is obvious, and in hospital practice this may be a decisive factor. Work with an individual patient will ensure a closer rapport and permit a more detailed study of the patient's needs.

We always have an introductory meeting with the group or the individual patient during which the whole programme of preparation is discussed and the patient's acceptance ensured. Frequently misunderstandings have to be dispelled. The patients then come confidently for the first session. This session is usually scheduled during the seventh month of pregnancy, and it is then that the patient's hypnotic capacity and behaviour are studied. The first hypnosis also helps to show the patient that there is no reason to fear losing his independence during the trance state. Regular weekly sessions of about a half hour are begun in the eighth month. During these sessions elementary knowledge is also conveyed concerning childbirth. Technical details are explained and all potentially harmful misconceptions eliminated.

When possible, hypnosis is deepened in the successive sessions and appropriate post-hypnotic suggestions are given. It is only after four or five sessions that a deep enough relaxation is usually reached. The patient is taught to relax each part of his body separately and to contract the various muscle groups at will. During the actual confinement this capacity will help to ensure better oxygenation of the tissues and alleviate spastic muscular contractions and the accompanying pain sensations. It also increases the woman's confidence in her active participation. Later on, autohypnosis is taught, and eventually combined with self-induced analgesia, the final step in the preparation.

It has been our experience that in groups of eight to ten women, it is a good thing, after preliminary exercises in relaxation, to have each woman go through an imaginary confinement. In groups, mutual influence of the participants plays a great role. Here it is our role to prepare patients to enter the confinement relaxed and confident rather than in a deep state of hypnosis.

With individualized preparation we have achieved the following results with one hundred consecutive patients:

Complete absence of pain, excellent cooperation of patient, no excitement	45
Excellent cooperation, no excitement, but pains felt at the end of the expulsion period	34
Fair results	12
Failures	9

Guéguen: I agree with most of the things just said. In most of my own cases, preparatory sessions are started in the sixth or seventh month, one of the reasons being that women are familiar with the psychoprophylactic method and expect such preparation. Nevertheless, it is one of the advantages of the hypnotic method that it can occasionally be used effectively without prior preparation. In that case, the woman is first hypnotized when she is admitted to the hospital. Whether she has had previous preparation or not, hypnosis is induced or reinduced at the beginning of labour, preferably before contractions have become painful. It is maintained until the head and shoulders of the child are born, then the trance is terminated in order to enable the woman to witness the rest of the birth in her normal waking state.

Unless the woman has been able to learn self-hypnosis, contact with the hypnotist must remain frequent during the confinement. In my experience as an obstetrician using hypnosis, I have found that my presence was more frequently required during the birth. In a limited number of cases, training in hypnosis during pregnancy was accomplished by another physician and the hypnotic rapport switched to me. This has meant an economy of time for the obstetrician and was quite satisfactory in its results.

We have always included in our hypnotic formulations suggestions to the effect that the parturiant woman would be able to hear and carry out orders given by the midwife or other attendants, and also that she should terminate the trance state by herself if need be. These were considered precautionary measures, since, practically speaking, constant presence of the hypnotist cannot be assured during the long hours of labour.

We have tried to have one of the midwives act as a hypnotist, or to switch the hypnotic rapport to her, but without much success.

As to the effects of hypnosis on labour and confinement, we have noted no unfavourable effect of hypnoanalgesia on the infant. Nor has it any effect on the quality of the uterine contractions or on the dilation of the cervix. The expulsion period is usually shortened. There is no greater frequency of obstetrical operations, forceps deliveries, episiotomies, etcetera. Such operations can be done under hypnotic anesthesia.

Results concerning pain relief have been the following: complete analgesia: 65%; satisfactory but incomplete analgesia: 18%; failure: 17%.

Völgyesi: We have distinguished between psychopassive and psychoactive individuals. The former are easily recognized by their inhibited and gauche attitude, vasomotor instability, and clammy hands. In these cases hypnosis can be induced rapidly and easily, and painlessness can be achieved almost immediately. In about one-fifth of the patients in this category, hypnotic analgesia will make childbirth as well as eventual instrumentation absolutely painless. In about two-thirds of the cases satisfactory analgesia can be achieved by combining with hypnosis very small doses of sedatives or narcotics. In our experience, patients requiring chemo-anesthesia should not exceed 10 to 15%.

Chairman: Dr. GUÉGUEN's remark concerning the failure of midwives as hypnotists opens an interesting avenue of study. In France, the training sessions required by the psychoprophylactic method are usually conducted by midwives. It has been my experience that one can frequently notice a kind of amazonish trait in these midwives, who are always urging their patients to greater efforts in order to achieve natural childbirth. If they succeed, they outdo the men, be they the father of the child or the obstetrician. Maybe that is why the father of the child is asked to be present at the birth, sheepish as he may feel and look. Before this method was introduced, a certain sisterly roughness seems to have been the prevalent attitude among midwives. If these observations are well founded, one can understand why the midwives would not feel at ease in the role which would become theirs in the use of hypnosis.

Hypnosis in childbirth is only one of its many applications we are considering today. I would now like to ask Dr. WOODWARD about its effect on the post-operative neuro-endocrine response.

C) Hypnosis and the neuro-endocrine response

Woodward: To deal with a calm and quiet patient for the induction of anesthesia is the aim of all pre-operative preparation. To achieve this end, hypnosis may be useful in certain cases, though obviously many others can do without it. Anxiety and fears of various natures produce most noxious effects at the time of induction of anesthesia. By reducing or abolishing fear, hypnosis acts as a de-alerting mechanism, avoiding the undesirable defence reactions. Its effects include limitation of adrenalin secretion, reduction of sweating, decreased motor activity, slowing of the pulse rate and lowering of the blood pressure. It is also said that ACTH secretion is lessened and adrenal-cortical secretion more nearly normal, both in quantity and in quality. This is related, among other things, to the healing of wounds, which usually proceeds in a very satisfactory manner among patients who have been hypnotized. The metabolic rate stays low in the hypnotized patient so that oxygen consumption is not increased. One of the most striking and dramatic effects of hypnosis is that of reduced bleeding during operation, which is due partly to the lowered blood pressure and partly to peripheral or localized vasoconstriction.

As I mentioned earlier, anesthetists want patients to be quiet before an operation. Also, a quiet, hypnotized patient who is still conscious will have a considerable effect on the anesthetist as well as on the surgeon or dentist. Their attitude will also become relaxed, and their behaviour will be reflected in the more adequate responses of the patient.

Hypnosis can be combined with chemo-anesthesia in still another way. During anesthetic induction as well as during emergence, in other words during every phase of very light anesthesia, verbal suggestions seem to be very effective. Under specific circumstances, like those we are familiar with in dental surgery under nitrous oxide, such a combination of a chemical with hypnotic suggestions can be easily put to good use.

Chairman: We are going to speak about dental anesthesia in a few moments. It might be of interest to mention here the various electrophysiologic studies on consciousness initiated by MAGOUN, and particularly the very important contributions made by Professor MARY A. B. BRAZIER on the mode of action of anesthetics with regard to consciousness. Three different functional components seem to be involved in consciousness: those necessary for the transmission of stimuli, those involved in the awareness of arrival of stimuli, and those responsible for keeping a memory of this arrival. With the help of modern electronic devices it has become possible to register the evoked potentials in various parts of the brain following specific sensory stimulations. It has been shown that the evoked cortical responses to visual and auditory stimuli are increased during light anesthesia. This concerns essentially the primary response to a stimulus reaching the cortex by way of the specific thalamic nucleus. The secondary waves appearing normally in the cortical region as a consequence of nerve impulses, mediated by the non-specific reticular system, are strongly depressed under anesthesia. So is the hippocampus, the formation Mrs. BRAZIER considers to be of prime importance in relation to memory.

One should also mention here the most interesting work of DAVID B. CHEEK demonstrating the possibility of recovering under hypnosis, with the help of the so-called ideomotor questioning technique, memories of events that occurred while the subject was under the influence of chemo-anesthesia. CHEEK stresses the dire consequences of provoking, by thoughtless remarks, dangerous reactions in the patient, such as hemorrhage, anuria, and so forth. Conversely, appropriate suggestions by the anesthetist could also have potent effects. The importance of what a patient "hears" during an operation under general anesthesia is obvious, and implies that a very strict discipline should be imposed on the whole surgical team. CHEEK's finding also involves the neurophysiology of hypnosis. According to PAVLOV's theory, anesthetics and hypnosis act by depressing the cerebral cortex. Now it seems to be more appropriate to study the ascending reticular formation and the hippocampus rather than the cortex.

Let us now continue our debate and ask Dr. GOLDIE to tell us about his experience with hypnosis in emergency operations.

D) Hypnosis in emergency operations

Goldie: An operative procedure requiring an anesthetic is in itself conducive to a high degree of suggestibility. Terms such as susceptibility and depth of hypnosis are misleading unless reference is made to the state and circumstances of the patient. Emergency operations are to be placed high on the list of situations increasing suggestibility. In these circumstances profound effects of psychological factors on physical processes can be demonstrated. Emergency operations present one of the few occasions when it may be justified to use suggestion as an aid to anesthesia or as a substitute for it, though precautions should be taken to ensure that conventional anesthesia will not be precluded should hypnosis fail.

The anesthetist has a special responsibility because he is in the best position in the surgical team to allay fears and contradict by reason the fantasies of the patient. Obviously, he has enough to do without becoming, in addition to an anesthetist, a psychiatrist, but there is every justification for studying the special nature of the situation in which he works, as it affects the physical preparation and recovery of the patient. If an emergency operation has to be performed, then clearly the operation takes precedence over any concern for psychological subtleties and sequelae. The anesthetist should therefore know enough to be able to utilize the psychological nature of the situation to facilitate the operation. Alternatively, if he is aware of the power he controls and uses it wisely, he can employ his knowledge of psychological factors for the immediate and long-term benefit of the patient in less urgent situations.

I would therefore advocate the procedure that I came to use when I practised hypnosis in the emergency theatre. The term hypnosis is unnecessary, and because of its lay connotations is best avoided. If asked, one should in all honesty be able to say that the patient's own resources are being used to help him. His and your experience show that this is possible, enabling an operation to be performed even though the patient has just had a large meal, eliminating the possibility of post-operative vomiting and reducing the time needed for recovery. The patient should know that he will come to no harm if this approach fails, and if recourse is had to an anesthetic. He should not fear that in this event he will be committed to standing great pain. The anesthetist should be prepared to use chemical anesthetics if necessary, and the surgeon should proceed without fear of eliciting pain. When an anesthetic has to be given, the psychological alleviation of anxiety can reduce the amount needed and reduce the risk of post-operative complications.

It is a great help if the anesthetist is relaxed as well as the patient; this is unlikely to be the case if he is self-consciously using a recipe that offends reason. But with a real understanding of the mental mechanisms involved in hypnosis he can feel that he is making use of ubiquitous mental mechanisms already experienced by the patient, and therefore that he is using a medical rather than an esoteric art. Informal discussion may reveal some sources of anxiety that he can allay and give him an indication of the way the patient is going to react. In my experience with acute minor surgery, there was a total absence of the severe anxiety reactions that I later described in my paper on "Spontaneous Traumatic Reactions to Hypnosis." Nevertheless, the anesthetist must beware of being seduced, along with the patient, into setting himself up as a magician or an omnipotent figure, an error to which hypnotists are prone.

To anesthetists schooled to look for "signs," "levels" and "stages," the procedure may seem particularly difficult as there is no consistency similar to that which he can expect in chemical anesthesia. In fact, the "stages" described by hypnotists in this situation are positively misleading. Analgesia is achieved, as in normal life, by obliviousness to certain sensations when mentally preoccupied. This is physiological or psychological fact. The patient, if agreeable, may be led to facilitate this process by several of the alternative means proposed by the anesthetist. Choosing appropriate words, this can be done more easily with children than with adults. Both doctor and patient should feel uncommitted, so that the doctor is able to say that this or that *may* happen, thus being truthful in suggesting to the patient possibilities that may be explored. If the desired result is not achieved this will lessen feelings of guilt and embarrassment, especially in the doctor.

Finally, the anesthetist should make it plain that hypnosis is not a panacea. The patient who has had an operation without chemical anesthesia may be impressed by the reality of psychological forces and consequently feel that this is also an easy way of dealing with psychological troubles. This is not the case, and hypnosis is of little value as an aid to psychological treatment.

Chairman: I think we all agree with one principle just stated by Dr. GOLDIE: in order to help the patient we want to enable him to use his own resources. For the sake of our fellow anesthetists we want to make it clear that such resources do exist and can be efficiently tapped. It happens that the ways and means to achieve this are quite outside the usual field of interest of the present-day anesthetist.

Dr. GOLDIE has certainly acted wisely in avoiding the term hypnosis in the emergency theatre. I wish we could do so under many other circumstances—maybe even here—in order to avoid mistaken connotations. One of these is the belief, on the part of both patient and doctor, that hypnosis is some kind of magic.

Goldie: A doctor who follows one of the simple rituals that used to be advocated for hypnosis may, in the right situation, send someone into an apparent hypnotic state without insight into what he is doing. Another may accomplish as much by using real psychological knowledge, thus making the experience one from which the patient may derive permanent benefit.

Many may have come to this symposium believing hypnosis to be something like an anesthetic, with techniques that can be described and with observable signs of different levels of consciousness. Unfortunately, it does not lend itself to such descriptions, since it is a psychological situation in which two people degenerate into an uncritical acceptance of each other's behaviour, implicitly taking this behaviour to indicate a belief in magic. That this psychological situation can have a profound effect on pain sensitivity was demonstrated by ESDAILE in the last century: he did more major operations using suggestion than anybody has before or since. But he never did the induction himself. He was a Mesmerist, and, as he believed that there was a vital substance involved that passed from one person to another, he had his patients "prepared" by Indian orderlies who spent hours passing their hands over patients before operation. If one wanted to learn the most successful technique then perhaps one should copy him, since, in a sense, he was the most successful of all hypnotists! However, we should not deride his "technique" before comparing it with the fantastic manoeuvres of some present-day hypnotists.

Three factors prevented medicine from learning from his experience: prejudice, his mistaken theory (Animal Magnetism) and the advent of chemical anesthetics. ESDAILE did hundreds of major operations, and judging by the fuss that is made today over odd operations done under hypnosis, we seem to have gone backwards, not forwards, in our psychological knowledge. The involved techniques shown in films of these operations make one wonder at the profound effects of hypnosis on hypnotists rather than on their patients. More recently, SHARPEY-SHAFER demonstrated that, in the case of chemical anesthesia for dental operations, the patients were going unconscious due to psychological factors, and were in some cases collapsing due to a fall in cardiac output before the mask touched the face! And this was described as a quiet anesthetic! A surgeon with whom I worked carried out major operations under local anesthesia, and during gastrectomies and thyroid operations at which I assisted patients frequently fell asleep, only to awaken immediately when the surgeon said that he had finished. There was no question of hypnosis, and anesthetists should therefore realize that what they do without hypnosis has suggestive properties. Many anesthetists have had the experience of one of my colleagues, who gave a child what he thought was an uneventful anesthetic only to discover later that he had not been delivering anesthetic gas to the patient. The situation had produced the desired effect.

Raginsky: While I agree with Dr. GOLDIE that hypnosis is certainly no panacea, I do not share his view concerning its value in psychotherapy. Far from being of little value, hypnosis in its various modern applications offers great possibilities, precisely by helping the patient to gain insight. My own experience with the method which I have called sensory hypnoplasty is ample proof of this contention.

Marmer: I want to take exception to Dr. GOLDIE's statement according to which hypnosis constitutes a psychological situation where people degenerate into an uncritical acceptance of each other's behaviour, both believing that some kind of magic is being practised. I consider this a definite misinterpretation of the situation, and it is contradicted by Dr. GOLDIE's own description of his actual handling of patients in the emergency theatre.

Stokvis: It is very difficult to make general statements concerning the value of any psychotherapeutic technique. In order to assess the results of various techniques, random distribution of patients to therapists and random use of therapeutic methods would be necessary. But in psychotherapy such randomization can never be achieved, and experiments along the line of the double blind arrangement are inherently impossible. Yet another difficulty lies in the definition of success in psychotherapy.

We have been using hypnosis in our clinic for more than thirty years. We go on using it, which shows that we consider it valuable, yet we are not overenthusiastic. We have tried to the best of our ability to assess the results of our therapeutic endeavours. We have found one-third of our patients free of complaints, one-third felt or seemed better, and the last third's condition remained unchanged or became worse. These figures were found whatever kind of psychotherapy had been used, whether hypnotic or not, and even in those cases where the initial consultation was followed by no psychotherapy whatsoever. I therefore feel that we should be extremely cautious in statements concerning therapeutic effects.

Chairman: Let us come back to the use of hypnosis in the various fields of surgery. I would first like Professor ZWICKER to comment on its role in general surgery.

Zwicker: We all agreed a short while ago on the fact that hypnosis cannot and should not compete with general anesthesia achieved by chemical means. On the other hand, it is my conviction that there is no method that can compete with hypnosis as a means to make an operation easy and its follow-up smooth. I do not feel that there is such a great difference between the patient's reactions and needs in the emergency situations described by Dr. GOLDIE and the majority of patients undergoing elective surgery. In the latter case the patients' fears of cancer, for instance, are greater in a gastric resection than in the reduction of a fracture incurred in some accident. Maybe the situation is different in more specialized fields of surgery.

Chairman: The department of anesthesiology of the University Hospitals in Mainz, Germany, directed by Professor R. FREY, is, to my knowledge, the only institution of its kind whose staff includes a psychologist active in hypnotherapy. In this capacity, T. VÁNDOR has been doing hypnotic psychotherapy principally with patients of the ear-nose-throat department, directed by Professor Dr. H. LEICHER. Perhaps he will now tell us about his experiences.

E) Hypnosis in E.N.T. surgery

Vándor: The aim of psychotherapy in surgery is to prevent or treat neurotic or psychotic reactions observed before or after accidents or operations. In the E.N.T. clinic, such reactions are seen mainly in the aftermath of operations affecting the capacity to hear or to speak, and after accidents or operations producing a change or deformity of the facial contour.

Psychosomatic therapy opens up a different field, less specific of E.N.T. surgery: the treatment of deranged autonomic functions (respiration, circulation or digestion) in the pre- and post-operative periods.

Finally, there is psychosomatic anesthesia, which includes the various combinations of suggestions, hypnosis, narcotics, and anesthetics, both general and local. We have found this combination useful to diminish fear and tension and to avoid or alleviate pain. During endoscopies, the combination of hypnosis with local spray reduces reflex activity. During throat surgery serious autonomic disturbances can be avoided, and the patient's fears of suffocating in his own blood during the operation can be effectively allayed.

In my belief, there is a special need for psychological preparation for tonsillectomies. The traumatic effect of an anesthetic which is not pleasant to inhale, to say the least, of being handled roughly, and of being operated on when the anesthetic effect has already worn off cannot be underestimated. After many other investigators, G. BIERMANN has recently given impressive proof of this contention. He asked children to make a drawing representing the operation. In the majority of cases these drawings depicted the surgeon as a monster.

Whenever circumstances permit preparing the patient for the operation, several sessions of hypnosis are in order. They usually start with simple relaxation, and deeper levels of hypnosis are attempted later. Occasionally a kind of rehearsal of the operation is staged, eventually including the manipulation of instruments. We also include everything pertaining to the anesthesia, be it local or general.

The situation is quite different when we meet the patient only shortly before the operation. Most of the time the patient is either tense or agitated, and mild, smoothing suggestions are then of no avail. It has been our experience that under such circumstances authoritative suggestions alone are effective in controlling the anxiety.

As with all other methods of anesthesia, the technique of psychosomatic anesthesia must always be adapted to the type of surgery and to the various phases of the operation. Let us take as an example the tonsillectomies already mentioned. Prior to, and at the beginning of the operation, we aim at quieting the patient and reducing his proneness to pain. Suggestions are concentrated on relaxation. It would be a mistake to continue these suggestions at the end of the operation, since surgical manipulation in the throat results in vagal stimulation. The patient is therefore prone to hypotension. On the other hand, the sight of blood or a vaso-vagal reflex can both end in loss of consciousness through a sudden drop in blood pressure. At this stage, therefore, we aim our suggestions towards a return of tension and muscular contraction. We also suggest deep breathing. If there is excessive bleeding, we suggest local cold on the throat so that the bleeding will be diminished without a drop in blood pressure. The practice of psychosomatic anesthesia cannot be restricted to the relationship between the patient and the anesthetist. It becomes the anesthetist's duty to prevent the patient from being harmed by the inappropriate surroundings frequently found in E.N.T. clinics. To expose children, just before the operation, to the sight of their comrades crying and spitting blood, or even to the noise of instruments being carried back and forth, is poor practice.

In our experience, two kinds of reaction can be observed as a consequence of psychic trauma induced by operations. In the first one, fear and pain are followed by an increased muscular tonus resulting in rigidity or excessive motor activity. In the second one, the experience of losing blood, most frequently induced when the patient sees, tastes, or swallows his own blood, and occasionally when he sees another person bleed, consists in a vasomotor reaction with hypotension and occasionally fainting.

We have been impressed by the difficulty of inducing and maintaining deeper levels of hypnosis for operations on the throat because of the defence reflexes. Waking suggestions, on the other hand, are frequently effective in these circumstances, and constitute a useful complement of the anesthetic.

In patients who are very hard of hearing, verbal suggestions are difficult or impossible to use.

Chairman: I would like to refer to a study done a few years ago in France by CAMPAN showing an average regression of mental age of about six months in children after tonsillectomy. The very unsatisfactory practice of short-inhalation anesthesia, which still prevails in most continental countries for tonsillectomies done on children held up in a sitting position, accounts for this. Proper anesthesia, with or without intubation, obliges the surgeon to change his habits and operate on a child in a supine position. In France, at least, resistance to this change has been very strong. If the anesthetist, by utilizing hypnosis, can improve matters until such time as the change is accomplished, he will certainly render great service to the patients.

Dr. VÁNDOR's observation of the favourable effects obtained by suggesting muscle contraction when a drop in blood pressure is to be feared opens an interesting field for hypnotherapy in surgery.

F) Hypnosis for hypothermia

Marmer: The use of hypothermia in cardiac surgery has brought about a great number of new problems. Various methods have been developed to lower the body temperature. Whenever this is done by exposing the body to a cold environment, shivering occurs unless the patient is anesthetized or paralyzed by curare. Chlorpromazine has also been used to prevent shivering, but this drug produces tachycardia and hypotension, which may constitute a dangerous stress for the patient's already severely burdened circulation. Unfortunately, all drugs used remain in the body for a more or less protracted period, and their effects can become excessive once the body temperature is lowered. Most anesthetists have therefore given preference to inhalation agents, in the hope of having these more rapidly eliminated from the system.

We have been able to show that shivering can be prevented under hypnosis by having an ice bath experienced by the patient as a pleasantly cool environment. With this method the use of drugs that are potentially dangerous in the hypothermal period can be dispensed with.

G) Hypnosis in dental surgery

Chairman: Let us switch from the highly specialized field of cardiac surgery to the more common practice of dental surgery. On the continent this is done mostly under local anesthesia, while in England general anesthesia is not infrequently used. I would like to ask Dr. WOODWARD to comment first of all on the latter.

Woodward: In most dental clinics in our country general anesthesia is used for both extractions and repair work. Much more dental care can be given in one sitting under general anesthesia than otherwise. The agent most commonly used is nitrous oxide because of its low toxicity, rapid action and elimination, and the absence of an explosion hazard. Unfortunately this agent also has its shortcomings. There may be excitement both during the induction phase and during maintenance. There is general agreement on the fact that at least 20% oxygen must be given to prevent anoxia, but unfortunately 80% nitrous oxide may be too weak to achieve general anesthesia. As BURNE has been able to show, this is constantly observed in patients who are used to drinking alcoholic beverages or who habitually take barbiturates as sleeping pills. Increased excitement or insufficient anesthesia will also result from psychological objections to general anesthesia on the part of the patient.

By preparing the patient for general anesthesia by the use of hypnotic suggestions, or by proceeding pari-passu with a hypnotic and a nitrous oxide induction, motor activity and oxygen consumption can be decreased and the anesthetic effect enhanced. Such a procedure will be effective regardless of the patient's habituation.

We have found this most advantageous when dealing with a nervous, tense and apprehensive patient, especially with children, young people, and those who have had a previous frightening experience with dentistry. We have been favourably impressed by the quiet recovery on emergence from the general anesthetic state, especially when the patient has been brought back to normal consciousness via a hypnotic state.

Stern: The use of hypnosis in dentistry is actually more widespread in the Anglo-Saxon countries than anywhere else. Perhaps the main reason for this strange fact lies in the predominantly pragmatic attitude in these countries which favours intellectual simplification. Such an attitude makes it easier for the dentist to use hypnosis and for the patient to experience it effectively. The initial aim of hypnodontia is to eliminate pain in dental operations. This hypnotic anesthesia or analgesia, with its freedom from anatomical innervation, is still one of the most impressive elements of hypnosis. To our knowledge, as practised in Europe today, hypnosis aims less at anesthesia than at the establishment of a good doctor-patient relationship by easing the patient's pre-operative fears.

Dental surgery has its own problems stemming from the poor visibility of the operative field and the uncomfortable position imposed on the surgeon. Reflex and defence movements of the patient can increase the difficulties to such an extent as to exhaust the operator or to make the operation nearly impossible. Means to reduce these are therefore of greatest interest to the dentist. Hypnotic suggestion can produce a relaxed mental and physical state that enables the patient to tolerate manipulations without being bothered or tired out. Of even greater importance is the action of hypnotic suggestion on salivation, gagging, coughing and fainting, since these are not of the patient's volition. When patients experience difficulty in tolerating dentures or other apparatus, in spite of proper fitting, post-hypnotic suggestions may be used.

Most effects of the latter type need medium or deep hypnosis, which can be achieved in most patients only after several sessions. In private practice in Europe, such preparation can be accomplished only in exceptional cases. Yet, with simple suggestions of relaxation, good results can be achieved without too much effort on the part of the practitioner. It is not easy for the dentist who is busy with the actual dental care to also watch his patient and adjust his suggestions accordingly. Instead of inducing a trance state and maintaining the patient in hypnosis during surgery, I have adopted a compromise solution which I have called psychosomatic premedication. Before starting surgery, I have the patient go through a certain number of exercises in relaxation, drawing his attention to his muscles and respiration. Such relaxation seems to increase pain tolerance while at the same time eliminating pain expectancy, since the patient's attention is focussed on a different bodily phenomenon.

Difficulties and dangers

Chairman: This panel is composed of men who are using hypnosis. Their conviction as to its usefulness can therefore be taken for granted. Instead of multiplying examples of how hypnosis can be used, it would be valuable for all of us and for our audience to hear about the difficulties encountered in practising hypnosis and the dangers its use could entail. I would like Dr. STOKVIS to speak first about the difficulties.

Stokvis: I intend to limit my remarks to difficulties in the induction of hypnosis. These can stem from the patient, the doctor, or a mistaken technique. These three factors are intimately interwoven, and it is only for the sake of clarity that we will consider them separately.

Let us begin with patient resistance. It may occasionally prevent hypnosis out of sheer misunderstanding. The need for adequate explanation is obvious if we think how frequently hypnosis is considered to imply giving over one's entire being into the control of the operator. A full explanation forms an essential part of the indispensable preliminary contact between patient and doctor. When hypnosis is used in a therapeutic context, the patient's acceptance of the eventual success of the therapy must be ensured. Since, in anesthesiology, the problem of pain is foremost, one must first establish how the patient experiences pain before submitting him to hypnotic treatment. In some patients severe pain may signify punishment and serve to relieve feelings of anxiety or guilt. Such a patient will resist suggestions as to the disappearance of his pain. Occasionally he may trade one symptom for another, but when finally deprived of his neurotic solution his anxiety will be freed and may turn into most undesirable manifestations, including an attempt to commit suicide.

A special form of resistance against hypnosis, found in highly suggestible personalities, consists in a negativistic attitude. Conscious of their weakness, these people resist out of fear. Though they believe that they act of their own free will, they are definitely under the influence of suggestion. But instead of accepting the suggestions uncritically, they reject them just as uncritically. Appropriate induction methods can circumvent this difficulty. In a more conscious way, resistance can take the form of various claims the patient may make even before the start of induction. He may state that he is too well-informed, too much of an individualist, or too strong-willed. These arguments may be merely misconceptions that are easily dispelled, or a façade for deep-rooted fear of being overpowered and reduced to helplessness.

Once induction has been started, resistance may take the form of a refusal to cooperate, going so far as to negate the experience of physiological phenomena such as the appearance of the contrasting colours in our induction method. The resistance therefore achieves an effective autosuggestion negating actual experience. To discover resistance during hypnosis requires careful observation of fine cues: the patient's withdrawal movement when the physician attempts to take the pulse, for example. Discussing the hypnotic experience after the session may also be helpful.

If we now consider the physician, we find that most difficulties will stem from his inhibitions. Whenever there is doubt in the physician about the procedure, he will be insecure, and his anxiety will contaminate the patient. Technical mistakes are frequently made because of such inner difficulties. I remember a young colleague who felt ridiculous in the middle of his first attempt to induce hypnosis. He thought that he had done nothing, stopped, and sent the patient away. The patient fell down the stairs. Another colleague succeeded in inducing hypnosis, but committed a very serious mistake. He left the patient, who appeared to be asleep, and forgot her. The patient refused to wake up when approached by others and had to be kept in the clinic overnight. Like resistance in the patient, resistance to hypnosis in the doctor can frequently be shown to be related to the transference situation involved. When the hypnotized patient (the child) notices insecurity in the hypnotist (the father or the mother), he will become anxious. This leads to the mistakes in technique that result in difficulties.

The preliminary interview must have given the physician information about the patient's transference situation. When the biography of a male patient shows arrest at the Oedipus situation, implying strong leaning towards the mother and hostility towards the father, identification of the hypnotist with the father will probably end up in failure. The hostile attitude towards the father will probably be transferred to the hypnotist, and the latter's suggestions will be opposed. Even in such circumstances a symptom can be removed because the patient, out of anxiety, would rather give up the symptom than stand the increased anxiety, accomplishing a sort of flight towards health.

Very strong positive transference can occasionally complicate a hypnotic treatment. The patient may experience this transference as a homosexual relationship and resist it as such. Here again, the physician must watch out and make sure he understands the transference situation.

Mistaken technique may increase certain fears concerning hypnosis in the patient. Some patients resist because they are afraid of coming under a magic influence, or of being submitted to narcosis, depriving them of contact with reality. Occasionally there are fears of being compelled to speak about or uncover hidden or forgotten memories. Sometimes the hypnotic situation will be associated with the feelings experienced in a former frightening situation, such as being raped. Here again, proper biographic investigation and information about the patient are necessary.

Stern: I would like to comment on Dr. STOKVIS' remarks in the perspective of the dental practitioner. Most of our patients' "knowledge" about hypnosis stems from some show they have seen in a music hall. It is therefore associated with the idea of fraud or with the belief in a special magical power. It is not easy to dispel these misconceptions. On the other hand, there are great differences in the behaviour of people of various nationalities when confronted by a person of authority. Some are used to accepting orders or even like being strongly disciplined. Such an attitude can be quite helpful when hypnosis is to be induced. Age, social standing, intellectual ability, general health, even the time of day may influence the outcome of a first hypnotic experience. When resistances of a psychological nature, conscious or unconscious, come into play, the time required to overcome this added difficulty may make hypnosis impossible to achieve within the limits imposed on the actual practice of dentistry. No doubt the practitioner's fame can be of great help, since many patients are already mentally prepared for hypnosis when they come for the first time. But the danger lies in having either to accept the role of a magician or to forego hypnosis in order to avoid being considered a charlatan.

There are other difficulties too. One can rightfully ask oneself whether a dentist's training enables him to make proper use of such a powerful psychotherapeutic tool as hypnosis. I quite agree that hypnosis properly practised hardly ever gives rise to serious difficulties. But the choice of suitable patients already requires a certain degree of psychological knowledge. It is not easy, with a dentist's approach to the patient, to make a differential diagnosis between neurosis, conversion hysteria or incipient psychosis. Finally, a good deal of attention to the patient's behaviour is necessary to induce hypnosis and to maintain it at a proper depth during the dental treatment. The dentist has therefore to divide his attention, and this exposes him to great strain. In my experience, this effort has been quite tiring, and all these various reasons have induced me to prefer what I have called psychosomatic premedication to actual hypnosis. A certain degree of relaxation can be induced even with standardized suggestions which are easily given and easily accepted.

Raginsky: How anybody uses hypnosis in his practice depends mainly on his concepts of it. If the physician is insecure and has a need to be powerful, dramatic or "different," he will most likely use it less effectively than one who is secure and obtains only the ordinary gratification from doing something well. In the latter instance there will be less need to use hypnosis as an "extraordinary activity," and it will become just another tool in the varied pool of techniques.

In the most sophisticated use of hypnosis there is less need to control the patient and to implant unnecessary suggestions. The more experienced and secure the hypnologist, the more he tends to use the hypnoidal state instead of deeper ones to obtain the same results. He is more apt to know when not to use hypnosis, and not to pursue it when all indications point to its minimal use.

Almost all patients can be helped to some degree through the use of the hypnoidal state alone. While it is not as impressive as deeper hypnotic states, nor as easily reported in literature, the anesthesiologist using this concept will nevertheless help more patients more consistently. With it, there is less danger of breaking down some valuable psychological defences it has taken years for the patient to erect. This attitude will also meet with more support and understanding on the part of the surgical staff, as the induction and recovery from anesthesia is made smoother and less dramatic. For best results, the anesthesiologist using hypnosis in his work should be familiar with the psychosomatic aspects of anesthesia and the essential psychodynamics of human behaviour.

Chairman: These difficulties raise the general question of the use of hypnosis. It seems appropriate to mention here the conclusions of a recent American study on this matter. The Council on Mental Health of the American Medical Association published a statement (JAMA Volume 180, No. 8 of May 26, 1962, page 693) which starts as follows: "There is a significant place for hypnosis in modern medical practice. In its 'Report on the Medical Use of Hypnosis' (JAMA Volume 168, September 13, 1958, pages 186 to 189), the American Medical Association has published the conclusions of its Council on Mental Health to this effect, reached after a two-year study of the subject. These conclusions were approved in 1958 by the Board of Trustees and the House of Delegates and therefore constitute the official policy of the AMA. They indicate that hypnotic techniques should be used within the scope of the professional training and competence of the physician or dentist who employs them; that a physician should use hypnosis in undertaking only such procedures as he would be qualified to undertake without it; that hypnosis should be used on a highly selective basis in accordance with specified indications and contraindications; that it should be used in association with other techniques, never becoming a single technique used under all circumstances by any physician; and that it should be employed only by professionally qualified individuals who have received proper training in its use."

The wisdom of not permitting hypnosis to be used as a substitute for some deficiency in a specific field of medicine is very obvious if we refer to its use in anesthesiology. Psychosomatic anesthesiology enlarges the scope of this specialty. There is additional knowledge to be acquired, but none of the old skills are to be forgotten. This brings up the question of how to acquire appropriate knowledge in hypnosis, a matter which has been thoroughly studied in the report just mentioned. It concludes that training in hypnosis should be based on an understanding of psychodynamics; that the trainee should undertake the treatment of a certain number of cases under supervision; that restrictions should be exercised in the selection of individuals for postgraduate training in hypnosis; and that such training would be needed at various levels. It is suggested that training should take one half to a full day per week for a period of nine to twelve months, with a minimum of 144 hours of study.

I believe most of us will agree to this, and also admit that such an extensive study constitutes, in a way, a difficulty, considering the already heavy schedule in the present-day training programme of anesthetists.

Marmer: I would like to stress a point just mentioned by Dr. LASSNER. It is most dangerous to use hypnosis when the anesthetist does not know anesthesiology. Hypnosis should be used only after one has mastered everything else in anesthesiology, and if this is the case, there are rare dangers and rare complications. An inadvertent spontaneous ab-reaction may occur as a random phenomenon, but if the anesthesiologist is psychologically oriented, and understands human psychodynamics, he will be able to recognize it and take care of it.

One of the difficulties with the use of hypnosis in anesthesia is that the other hospital personnel (nurses and doctors) usually do not know how to take care of these patients. Most of the difficulties which arise are due to mishandling and misunderstanding in the care of these patients.

The use of local anesthesia to infiltrate the skin in association with hypnoanesthesia is not unusual, nor is it to be considered a negation of the hypnotic technique. Why should it make any difference? Are we trying to achieve omnipotence? Hypnosis should be used neither as a treat nor as a treatment. It should be used when it is in the best interests of the patient, and when the patient, not the anesthetist, will derive the greatest benefit therefrom. Hypnosis when used as another anesthesiological modality will find its lasting place in the practice of our specialty.

Zwicker: Over the last twenty years I have induced hypnosis in several thousand patients and have yet to see any harm resulting from it. No doubt this requires experience in psychotherapy. But since we use hypnosis in the field of surgery this knowledge is not enough. Whether symptoms should be approached by psychotherapeutic methods alone, or whether some somatic treatment is needed as well can be judged only when the doctor in charge of the case has sufficient knowledge in those fields. Psychosomatic medicine can be practised only when we are familiar with the psychological and somatic aspects of disease. May I draw upon a case history as an example?

A patient was referred to me for psychotherapy by a colleague specializing in internal medicine. This middle-aged woman had been suffering for more than ten years from gastric troubles considered to be functional. Only once in the many X-ray studies a small ulcer had been found on the lesser curvature. Later X-ray studies had been interpreted as showing only a residual scarring. The patient's mother had died from carcinoma of the stomach, and the patient had a phobic fear of cancer. While the psychological disturbances in this patient were very obvious, the location of the ulcer, its persistance, and also the fact that gastric acidity was low induced us to suggest exploratory laparotomy. A gastric ulcer of benign appearance was found and a partial gastric resection done. The pathological

finding of malignant degeneration in a part of this ulcer came
to us as a complete surprise.

There should be no precedence of psychological considera-
tions over somatic ones or vice versa. They each exist in their
own right. Certainly many more mistakes are made in surgery
by underestimating psychological factors than by overestimating
them. Very frequently operations are done, and even organs
removed, because conversion symptoms are misinterpreted. One
of the best-known mistakes is the acceptance by the surgeon of
the pressing demand of a patient for some operation. Although
the psychological implications of this desire for an expiatory
bodily insult have been widely publicized, these patients, who
often already bear the scars of previous operations, nevertheless
nearly always succeed in finding a surgeon ready to comply.

Chairman: Dr. STOKVIS has brought out how the doctor's
personality and the patient's mental set-up and socio-economic
situation are intimately interwoven in producing a condition
that makes the induction of hypnosis easy or difficult. Dr. STERN
has illustrated one aspect of this, dwelling mainly on an authoritarian approach. Dr. RAGINSKY and Dr. MARMER have stressed
the advantages of the permissive approach, both living in
countries where the authoritarian approach is seldom appropriate. No doubt it would be best to find out each patient's
individual needs and learn to be able to act accordingly.

This has led us to mention the difficulties of learning how
to overcome one's own limitations. We all accept the fact that we
are better with some techniques than with others because we are
more experienced with, let's say, general anesthesia than with
spinal anesthesia, but we aim to overcome this limitation by
proper training. The limitations imposed by our own abilities or
inabilities are even more manifest in psychotherapy. It may even
be queried whether one can really overcome them, for the
tendency to reject a method one is not in agreement with, aided
by some rationalization which devaluates it, is ubiquitous. The
greatest difficulty arising from the introduction of any psychological method in the field of medicine stems from this necessity
to take the physician's intimate personality into account.

Professor ZWICKER's remarks have shown one potential
danger of a one-sided psychological approach. There are various

others, mainly with hypnosis, as Dr. GOLDIE has already pointed out in reference to its use with children. Maybe we can take up this point once more.

Finer: I would like to quote a "peripatetic correspondent's" letter which appeared in *The Lancet* in 1961.

"A consultant came across a small boy struggling with the chain of his bicycle, which had become disengaged from its sprockets. Good-naturedly he lent a hand, replaced the chain, and tightened it expertly by adjusting the back hub. 'There,' he said, 'that should be all right now. Of course I cannot absolutely promise that it will never happen again. Suppose you let me see it again in a month's time?' At the end of a month he exclaimed, 'Capital, capital,' beaming and striking the saddle three times with his pencil. 'No trouble? Capital. Let's see it again in another month's time.' And so it went on, but the small boy, fearful that his bicycle might fail him when far from home, lost all zest for cycling, and soon gave it up altogether. But he continued to take his machine to the consultant for quite a long time."

This story demonstrates how important it is that the patient understand from the beginning that he plays an active role in the treatment and in the results which follow. Once this understanding is achieved, there is little danger that the patient will assume a position of dependence or presume that symptoms will disappear by irrational means.

Raginsky: The danger of fostering an attitude of dependency is definitely greater with an authoritarian approach. At the same time this approach frequently antagonizes or browbeats the patient. Unless the physician is motivated by a need to hide his insecurity behind an appearance of being powerful, he will rarely find these dramatics useful.

Antitch: I would like to mention the medico-legal aspects of using hypnosis in anesthesiology. The courts have been concerned with the use and abuse of hypnosis in various countries, both in the past and in the present. It is easy for the anesthetist to obtain a patient's agreement to use hypnosis for the purpose of making surgery or the recovery from it painless or less dangerous and unpleasant. The threat of the coming operation makes the patient more susceptible to hypnosis, and the drugs used by the anesthetist exert a similar facilitating influence. But it is a well-known fact that it becomes progressively easier to induce hypnosis with each repetition. It may become possible to induce it by a signal, even without the hypnotized person's knowledge, or against his will. In this way, the initial legitimate use may pave the way to possible abuse. There is also the danger of choosing a signal for the induction of hypnosis which may be encountered fortuitously. For instance, a specific brilliant object used in the eye fixation method could be seen by the subject under circumstances where the production of a trance state could entail some form of danger to his integrity. In a similar way self-hypnosis, which is sometimes used for the production of analgesia, may become dangerous.

Obviously the fact of having been hypnotized once represents a danger, since repeated hypnosis is then possible. This renewed hypnosis not only exposes the individual to various accidents, but even constitutes the basis for eventual criminal acts on or by the hypnotized subject. There have been many experiments to demonstrate the latter possibility. I would like to point out a recent book on this topic: PAUL J. REITER's *Antisocial or Criminal Acts and Hypnosis* (Thomas, Springfield, 1959).

At the end of the last century BENTIVEGNI studied the importance of hypnosis in civil law. He distinguishes responsibility in business and liability for damages with respect to hypnosis. The first denotes "a degree of freedom of will necessary for the transaction of business in connection with legal affairs." Liability for damages depends on the freedom of will connected with responsibility for unlawful acts. According to the common law of a number of countries, liability for damage cannot be assumed when an agent is not in possession of his reason and is therefore not able to control his actions. Where consciousness is partly or wholly absent there can be no responsibility. There is one exception to this rule: the subject's request to be hypnotized or his assent to undergo hypnosis in order to avoid responsibility.

Another medico-legal aspect of hypnosis is its use to obtain so-called material truths. The use of such truths by the court would, in almost all circumstances, be contrary to the contents of the Universal Declaration of Human Rights and even with the contents of the Geneva Conventions.

In order to prevent possible abuse of hypnosis through the increased susceptibility to hypnosis after the first hypnotic induction, international regulations should be urgently made to restrict the use of hypnosis to medical treatment.

Chairman: There are rather easy technical means available to protect the patient against the spontaneous occurrence of a trance state or of its production by an unqualified operator. Dr. Antitch's timely reminder should bring about a reconsideration of the wisdom of transferring the hypnotic relationship to auxiliaries, as it has been done in obstetrics. On the whole, I think we are all in agreement that the practice of hypnosis should be restricted to physicians. Similar regulations are urgently needed in the field of anesthesiology as well. The practice of anesthesia should certainly be restricted to doctors only, and to doctors given appropriate training.

Schmid-Schmidsfelden: The dangers of medico-legal implications just mentioned should not be exaggerated. Nearly every treatment can be abused. Since it requires a special effort on the part of the anesthetist to use psychological methods, the scarecrow of law suits could definitely prevent him from entering this field.

What Dr. Stern said for the dentist holds true for the anesthetist too. Hypnosis needs time and patience, both of which are frequently lacking in our respective departments. It also needs learning, which in most countries has to be autodidactic. I would like to dwell at some length on the material difficulties encountered by the anesthetist who has nevertheless finally come to practise hypnosis. He will have to adopt a new time schedule, since most of us have to do clinical work in the operating room, give post-operative care both in the recovery room and in the surgical wards, do pre-operative visits, nerve-block therapy, etcetera. Another distinct difficulty lies in the architectural arrangement of most surgical wards and departments of anesthesia. There is hardly ever a room where the anesthetist can see his patient quietly and without disturbing the hospital routine. The present shortage of anesthetists the world over exposes all of us to overwork and to frequent calls when we are both in the hospital and outside of it. It is very hard to prevent disturbing calls during a psychotherapeutic session, and even harder to tolerate them.

The practice of hypnosis or other psychotherapy by the anesthetist arouses feelings of curiosity, if not of hostility, among fellow anesthetists, surgeons and nurses. It is also likely to disturb the patient's relatives. Obviously one has to obtain a child's parents' consent before using hypnosis. Some little explanation given to the patient's relatives and visitors may also be helpful. It would require a study in itself to analyze the reactions of the medical personnel. In the beginning, incomprehension, jealousy, derogatory remarks, indirect signs of hostility like slamming of doors, unnecessarily noisy calls, and so forth, are very frequent. Eventually, too much of a generally hostile atmosphere around the efforts of the newly-come or self-made psychologically-oriented anesthetist may prevent the success of his endeavour. An occasional patient may refuse hypnosis, despite all the explanations given, because he has been influenced by the negativistic attitude manifested by the other hospital personnel in contact with him. This situation may even undermine a man's confidence in the whole new approach he is attempting and prevent him from pursuing a worthwhile task.

Finer: The extension of the activities of the anesthetist into the field of psychotherapy definitely complicates his life. And it takes a long time before his abilities in this field are appreciated. For quite some time he will be the object of criticism from psychiatrists and surgeons as well as from his fellow anesthetists. Wherever his position is not one of independence but, as is so frequently the case in continental Europe, one of subordination to the head of the surgical department or to a board of hospital management, his interest in hypnosis may well jeopardize his professional career.

I feel that the definition of hypnosis as a state of heightened suggestibility—given by WEIZENHOFFER in 1953, and much in line with last century's thought as expressed by BERNHEIM—is a definite hindrance to its acceptance and understanding. Such a definition also fosters to a certain extent the hostile attitudes towards hypnosis, since suggestibility evokes the idea of credulity, and heightening it is easily interpreted as attempting some kind of fraud. I would much rather advocate calling hypnosis a state of learned concentration. Since we use the word doctor from the Latin *doceo*, meaning to teach, the teaching of learned concentration will easily be accepted as coming within the realm of the doctor. The patient should have no objections to being considered a pupil, nor to learning to concentrate in such a way as to achieve detachment from fear or pain.

Völgyesi: My records today include 55,000 patients whom I have hypnotized in over forty years of practice. The only harmful effects of hypnosis I have ever observed have resulted from its use by unqualified people: performers in music-hall shows, members of certain religious sects, and so forth. Whether to use the so-called authoritarian approach, which implies an immediate induction of hypnosis, or some slower psychotherapeutic technique can be easily determined by applying appropriate rules of typology. In people who show the characteristics of psychopassivity, and who also show hyperhypnophily, immediate hypnotization usually gives the best results.

We have to give up our former dominant interest in somatic diagnosis, and in every case consider the psychological factors to be of equal importance. Disease is a consequence of exogenous and endogenous stresses. Nature, society, and the patient's make-up are all in play to prevent or cure disease; therefore all must be considered. This is the aim of the movement I have started under the name The School of Patients. It can be considered as an extension of psychoprophylaxis, formerly applied only to childbirth, to all fields of medicine.

Stokvis: I have already indicated that although I constantly use hypnosis I consider it a mistake to be overenthusiastic about it. Overenthusiasm can easily lead to the use of this method for the benefit of the practitioner rather than for that of the patient. One cannot conceive of a treatment that would be appropriate for all patients. To act as if one were in possession of such a panacea and to employ it without a valid reason does not necessarily end up in damage to the patient, but it does not constitute appropriate care. I certainly share Dr. VÖLGYESI's view that consideration should be given to the psychological implications in every patient. This is the basic contention in our practice of psychosomatic medicine.

As to the danger of hypnosis, I also agree with Dr. VÖLGYESI that there is none as long as it is applied only in appropriate cases. The so-called addiction to hypnosis has hardly ever been observed, and it is certainly untrue that the hypnotized person could become entirely dependent on the hypnotist, like an automaton. As to side effects like somnolence, hallucinations, anxiety, vertigo and headaches, they appear only as a result of faulty techniques.

Conclusion

Chairman: The difficulties and dangers of hypnosis which have been mentioned can be avoided or overcome. In order to avoid them the user must have learned to master his relationship with the patient. He also has to understand his own tendency to use hypnosis or refuse it, and at the same time be able to distinguish whether its use is necessary or not. To do so, he will have to conduct a preliminary interview with the patient. It is an open question whether or not he should mention hypnosis by name during this interview. Should the interview lead him to fear inducing hypnosis, he should abstain. Should he nevertheless consider hypnosis appropriate, he should proceed with great caution. For the practice of anesthesiology, the change of orientation given to the pre-operative visit is of prime importance. The anesthetist has to become cognizant of the psychological implications of this visit and learn to use it accordingly.

Some members of this panel have expressed the hope that the anesthetist's professional status might be improved by broadening his scope to include psychotherapeutic measures in his practice. Others have voiced the fear that he might thus jeopardize whatever status he has already achieved. Both opinions are probably justified in their own right, since both events can happen. Which way the scale tips will depend essentially on what has been put in the balance to counteract the weight of prejudice and blind hostility.

It may be appropriate to conclude our debate on hypnosis by remembering with gratitude that we have been invited to hold it at this First European Congress of Anesthesiology in the very city of Vienna where, nearly two centuries ago, FRANZ ANTON MESMER discovered its possibilities in medicine. The deeper implications of the hostility aroused by it can be understood better today thanks to another physician whose name will forever be linked with the city of Vienna: SIGMUND FREUD, who himself encountered difficulties in many respects similar to those experienced by MESMER. Let us in our own smaller ways continue in their path.

GPSR Compliance

*The European Union's (EU) General Product Safety Regulation (GPSR)
is a set of rules that requires consumer products to be safe and our
obligations to ensure this.*

*If you have any concerns about our products, you can contact us on
ProductSafety@springernature.com*

In case Publisher is established outside the EU, the EU authorized
representative is:

Springer Nature Customer Service Center GmbH
Europaplatz 3
69115 Heidelberg, Germany

Batch number: 09635029

Printed by Printforce, the Netherlands